Hormone Reset Diet Recipes

Effective & Delicious Hormone Reset Recipes for Weight Loss & Health

By Kira Novac

ISBN: 978-1-80095-003-0

Copyright ©Kira Novac 2016

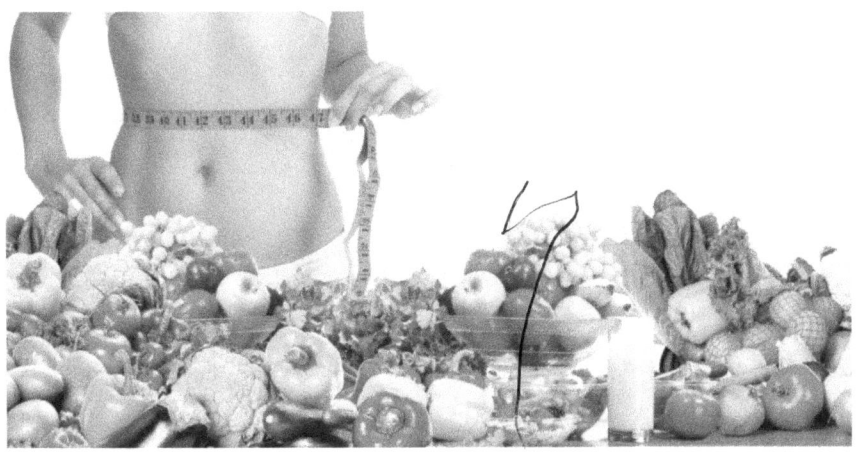

All rights reserved. No part of this publication may be reproduced, stored in a retrieval system, or transmitted, in any form or by any means, electronic, mechanical, photocopying, recording or otherwise, without the prior written permission of the author and the publishers.

The scanning, uploading, and distribution of this book via the Internet, or via any other means, without the permission of the author is illegal and punishable by law. Please purchase only authorized electronic editions, and do not participate in or encourage electronic piracy of copyrighted materials.

All information in this book has been carefully researched and checked for factual accuracy. However, the author and publishers make no warranty, expressed or implied, that the information contained herein is appropriate for every individual, situation or purpose, and assume no responsibility for errors or omission. The reader assumes the risk and full responsibility for all actions, and the author will not be held liable for any loss or damage, whether consequential, incidental, and special or otherwise, that may result from the information presented in this publication.

A physician has not written the information in this book. Before making any serious dietary changes, I advise you to consult with your physician first.

A GIFT TO MY READERS

Irresistible Gluten Free Desserts, Snacks & Treats

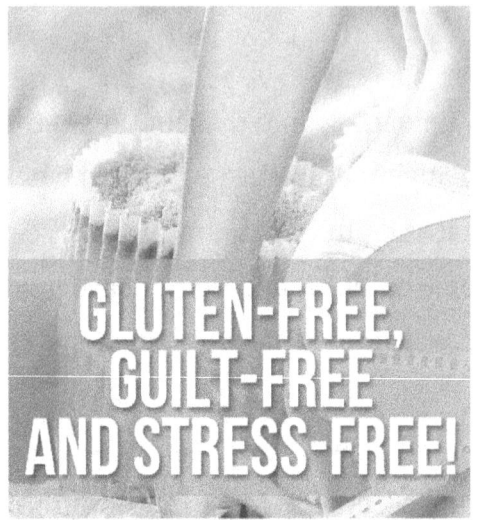

You can download your free recipe eBook at:

http://www.bit.ly/gluten-free-books

Now, let's jump into the recipes!

Table of Contents

Introduction 4
   Recipe Measurements 5
Hormone Reset Shakes and Beverages 6
   Avocado Walnut Lime Smoothie 6
   Mint Chocolate Chia Shake 7
   Simple Ginger Beet Juice 8
   Vanilla Almond Shake 9
   Homemade Detox Tea 10
   Easy Chocolate Protein Shake 11
   Kale, Dandelion and Carrot Juice 12
   Chocolate Hazelnut Shake 13
   Vanilla and Greens Smoothie 14
   Creamy Cashew Coconut Shake 15
   Cucumber Spinach Smoothie 16
   Coco-Almond Protein Shake 17
Hormone Reset Breakfast Recipes 19
   Spiced Pumpkin Porridge 19
   Mushroom Scallion Egg Muffins 20
   Nuts and Seeds Porridge 21
   Tomato Basil Omelet 23
   Maple Pecan Grain-Free Granola 24
   Broccoli Onion Egg Muffins 25
   Sweet Potato Cauliflower Hash 26
Hormone Reset Soups and Salads 27
   Warm Quinoa Veggie Salad 27

Dairy-Free Cream of Broccoli Soup 29
Cucumber, Red Onion, Dill Salad 31
Chilled Avocado Soup with Paprika 32
Dairy-Free Broccoli Salad 33
Creamy Butternut Squash Soup 35
Red Cabbage and Carrot Slaw 36
Hearty Curried Lentil Soup 37
Spinach Salad with Avocado and Chickpeas 38
Southwestern Chicken Soup 39

Hormone Reset Snacks and Sides 41

Baked Zucchini Fritters 41
Cocoa Cashew Butter Bars 42
Lemon Garlic Hummus 43
Sesame Kale Chips 44
Baked Sweet Potato Wedges 45
Roasted Red Pepper Hummus 46
Dairy-Free Basil Pesto 47
Baked Squash Fries 48
Spicy White Bean Hummus 49
Easy Chia Seed Pudding 50
Homemade Dairy-Free Cheese 51
Almond Butter Fudge Cups 52

Hormone Reset Main Entrees 53

Coconut-Crusted Halibut Fillets 53
Sweet Potato Chickpea Curry 54
Cajun-Style Seared Scallops 55
Zucchini Pasta with Lemon Sauce 56

Black Bean Mushroom Burgers 57
Gluten-Free Crab Cakes 58
Seared Swordfish with Salsa 59
Cilantro Herbed Turkey Burgers 60
Quick and Easy Ceviche 61
Balsamic Portabella Burgers 62
Spaghetti Squash with Sautéed Veggies 63

Conclusion **64**
DON'T FORGET YOUR FREE EBOOK **65**

Introduction

The human body is a complex machine with many individual parts that work together as a whole. Each and every day, your body produces a variety of different substances which spark and facilitate certain reactions. Hormones are a type of biochemical that affect the way your body and your mind works – they also play a role in combating stress, maintaining muscle tissue, and storing fat. If you are looking for a way to lose weight and improve your energy levels, balancing your hormones by following a hormone reset diet might be the secret trick you've been looking for.

A hormone reset diet should last about 21 days – that is how long researchers suggest it takes for something to become habit. During the 21 days of the diet you will systematically remove 7 key foods or food groups in 3-day bursts to reset your hormones. First you will give up meat and alcohol to help reset your estrogen levels. Next, give up sugar to help reset your body's insulin receptivity. Third, remove fruits to target your leptin, the hunger hormone. Next, give up caffeine to reset your body's response to stress and the stress hormone, cortisol. Fifth, go grain-free to activate your thyroid hormone then go dairy-free to reset your growth hormone. Finally, give up toxins to help reset testosterone levels while also supporting the reset of all other hormones.

Recipe Measurements

I love keeping ingredient measurements as simple as possible- this is why I stick to tablespoons, teaspoons and cups.

The cup measurement I use is the American cup measurement. I also use it for dry ingredients. If you are new to it, let me help you:

If you don't have American Cup measures, just use a metric or imperial liquid measuring jug and fill your jug with your ingredient to the corresponding level. Here's how to go about it:

1 American Cup= 250ml= 8 fl.oz

For example:

If a recipe calls for 1 cup of almonds, simply place your almonds into your measuring jug until it reaches the 250 ml/8oz mark.

I know that different countries use different measurements and I wanted to make things simple for you.

Hormone Reset Shakes and Beverages

Avocado Walnut Lime Smoothie
Servings: 1 to 2

Ingredients:

- 1 cup unsweetened almond milk
- ½ cup ice cubes
- 1 cup chopped kale or spinach
- ½ medium ripe avocado, pitted and chopped
- ¼ cup chopped walnuts
- 2 tablespoons fresh lime juice
- ½ teaspoon fresh lime zest

Instructions:

1. Place the spinach and avocado in a high-speed blender together.
2. Pour in your almond milk then blend the ingredients well.
3. Add in your other smoothie ingredients and then push the pulse button a few times.
4. Blend for about 30 to 45 seconds until the ingredients are smooth.
5. Pour your smoothie into a large glass to serve.

Mint Chocolate Chia Shake

Servings: 1 to 2

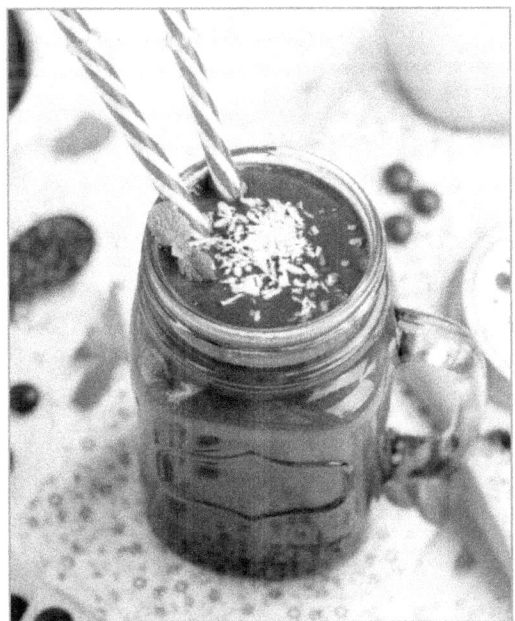

Ingredients:

- 1 ½ cups unsweetened almond milk
- ½ cup ice cubes
- 1 bunch fresh mint leaves
- 2 scoops chocolate protein powder
- ¼ cup raw cacao nibs

Instructions:

1. Combine all of your shake ingredients into a powerful blender.
2. Press the pulse button several times to chop the smoothie ingredients.
3. Blend the ingredients for about 30 to 45 seconds on the highest speed setting.
4. Once the shake is blended smooth, pour it into a glass to serve.

Simple Ginger Beet Juice

Servings: 1 to 2

Ingredients:

- 2 to 3 kale leaves, chopped
- 2 small carrots, peeled and diced
- 1 medium-sized beet, peeled and chopped
- 1 ½ cups water
- 1 tablespoon fresh minced ginger
- ½ cup ice cubes

Instructions:

1. Place the kale, carrot and beet in a high-speed blender together.
2. Pour in your water, ginger and your ice cubes and then blend up your ingredients.
3. Blend for about 30 to 45 seconds until the ingredients are smooth.
4. Cover a large glass with cheesecloth then pour the liquid through it.
5. Squeeze the cheesecloth, straining as much liquid into the glass as you can.
6. Serve the juice cold garnished with a slice of beet.

Vanilla Almond Shake
Servings: 1

Ingredients:

- 1 cup unsweetened coconut milk
- ½ cup ice cubes
- 2 scoops vanilla protein powder
- 2 tablespoons almond butter
- ¼ teaspoon vanilla extract

Instructions:

1. Combine all of your shake ingredients together in a high-speed blender.
2. Press the pulse button several times to chop the smoothie ingredients.
3. Blend the ingredients for about 30 to 45 seconds on the highest speed setting.
4. Once the shake is blended smooth, pour it into a glass to serve.

Homemade Detox Tea

Servings: 1 to 2

Ingredients:

- 1-inch fresh ginger, peeled
- 2 slices of fresh lemon
- 2 cups of water

Instructions:

1. Combine your ginger and your lemon in a small-sized pot along with your water.
2. Bring the mixture to simmering on the high heat setting.
3. Once it boils, lower the heat setting and then simmer your tea ingredients for 10 minutes.
4. Remove the saucepan from the stove and cool for 5 minutes.
5. Take the lemon and ginger out then pour into a mug to serve.

Easy Chocolate Protein Shake
Servings: 1

Ingredients:

- 1 cup unsweetened almond milk
- ½ cup ice cubes
- 2 scoops chocolate protein powder
- 2 tablespoons raw cacao nibs

Instructions:

1. Combine all of your shake ingredients together in a high-speed blender.
2. Press the pulse button several times to chop the smoothie ingredients.
3. Blend the ingredients for about 30 to 45 seconds on the highest speed setting.
4. Once the shake is blended smooth, pour it into a glass to serve.

Kale, Dandelion and Carrot Juice
Servings: 1 to 2

Ingredients:

- 1 cup of chopped fresh chopped kale
- 1 cup of fresh chopped dandelion greens
- 1 medium carrot, peeled and chopped
- 1 ½ cups of chilled water
- 2 tablespoons of fresh lemon juice

Instructions:

1. Place the kale, dandelion greens and carrot in a high-speed blender together.
2. Pour in your water and lemon juice then blend the ingredients well.
3. Blend for about 30 to 45 seconds until the ingredients are smooth.
4. Cover a large glass with cheesecloth then pour the liquid through it.
5. Squeeze the cheesecloth, straining as much liquid into the glass as you can.
6. Serve the juice cold garnished with a slice of carrot.

Chocolate Hazelnut Shake
Servings: 1

Ingredients:

- 1 cup unsweetened hazelnut milk
- ½ cup ice cubes
- 2 scoops chocolate protein powder
- 2 tablespoons cashew butter
- 1 tablespoon raw cacao nibs

Instructions:

1. Combine all of your shake ingredients together in a high-speed blender.
2. Press the pulse button several times to chop the smoothie ingredients.
3. Blend the ingredients for about 30 to 45 seconds on the highest speed setting.
4. Once the shake is blended smooth, pour it into a glass to serve.

Vanilla and Greens Smoothie

Servings: 1 to 2

Ingredients:

- 2 cups of fresh chopped spinach
- 1 small cucumber, peeled and chopped
- ¼ cup of fresh chopped parsley or cilantro
- 1 cup of chilled coconut water
- ½ cup of ice cubes
- ¼ teaspoon of vanilla extract

Instructions:

1. Place the spinach and your cucumber inside a powerful blender.
2. Pour in your coconut milk then blend the ingredients well.
3. Add the rest of the smoothie ingredients and pulse a few times.
4. Blend for about 30 to 45 seconds until the ingredients are smooth.
5. Pour your smoothie into a large glass to serve.

Creamy Cashew Coconut Shake
Servings: 1

Ingredients:

- 1 ½ cups unsweetened cashew milk
- 1 cup ice cubes
- 2 scoops vanilla protein powder
- ¼ cup unsweetened shredded coconut
- 1 tablespoon cashew butter

Instructions:

1. Combine all of your shake ingredients together in a high-speed blender.
2. Press the pulse button several times to chop the smoothie ingredients.
3. Blend the ingredients for about 30 to 45 seconds on the highest speed setting.
4. Once the shake is blended smooth, pour it into a glass to serve.

Cucumber Spinach Smoothie

Servings: 1 to 2

Ingredients:

- 1 ½ cups of fresh chopped spinach
- 1 small cucumber, peeled and chopped
- 1 cup of unsweetened almond milk
- ½ cup of ice cubes
- 1 tablespoon of raw chia seeds

Instructions:

1. Place the spinach and cucumber in a high-speed blender together.
2. Pour in your almond milk then blend the ingredients well.
3. Add in your ice cubes and chia seeds then blend for about 30 to 45 seconds until the ingredients are smooth.
4. Serve the smoothie cold garnished with a slice of cucumber.

Coco-Almond Protein Shake

Servings: 1

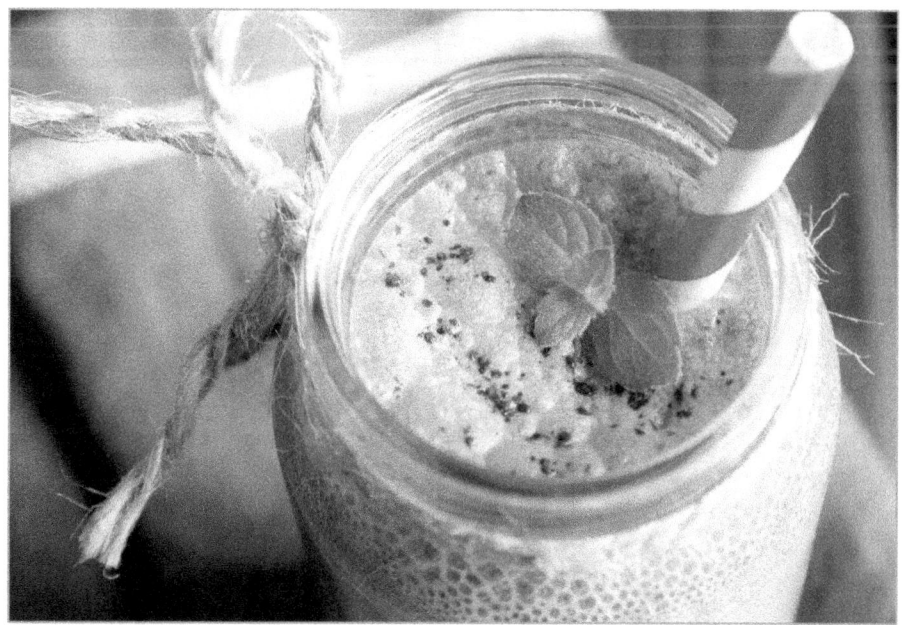

Ingredients:

- 1 cup unsweetened coconut milk
- ½ cup ice cubes
- 2 scoops vanilla protein powder
- 2 tablespoons sliced almonds
- 1 tablespoon of almond butter
- 1 tablespoon of raw cacao nibs

Instructions:

1. Combine all of your shake ingredients together in a high-speed blender.

2. Press the pulse button several times to chop the smoothie ingredients.
3. Blend the ingredients for about 30 to 45 seconds on the highest speed setting.
4. Once the shake is blended smooth, pour it into a glass to serve.

Hormone Reset Breakfast Recipes

Spiced Pumpkin Porridge
Servings: 4

Ingredients:

- 2 tablespoons of coconut oil
- 2 cups of canned pumpkin puree
- ½ to 1 cup of unsweetened almond milk
- ½ cup of ground flaxseeds
- ¼ cup of almond butter
- 1 ½ teaspoons of ground cinnamon
- ¼ teaspoon of ground nutmeg

Instructions:

1. Melt your coconut oil inside of a small saucepan on the low heat setting.
2. Stir in your pumpkin and almond milk.
3. Add in your flaxseed and your natural almond butter as well as the spices.
4. Cook the mixture, stirring it often, until it is heated through. Serve warm.

Mushroom Scallion Egg Muffins

Servings: 12

Ingredients:

- 1 teaspoon of coconut oil
- 2 cups of sliced mushrooms
- 1 clove of garlic, minced
- Pepper and salt as needed
- 12 large eggs, whisked well
- 2 scallions, sliced very thin

Instructions:

1. Preheat your oven to a temperature of 350°F.
2. Spray the 12 cups in a regular muffin pan with some cooking spray.
3. Melt your coconut oil into a skillet that has been heated on the medium-high heat setting.
4. Add in the mushrooms and garlic then season them with some pepper and salt.
5. Cook the mushrooms for 5 to 6 minutes until tender then take off the heat.
6. Spoon the cooked mushrooms into your prepared muffin pan evenly.
7. In a bowl stir thoroughly your eggs and scallions.
8. Pour the egg mixture into your muffin pan evenly then cook.
9. Cook them for 20 to 25 minutes until your egg muffins are completely set.

Nuts and Seeds Porridge

Servings: 4

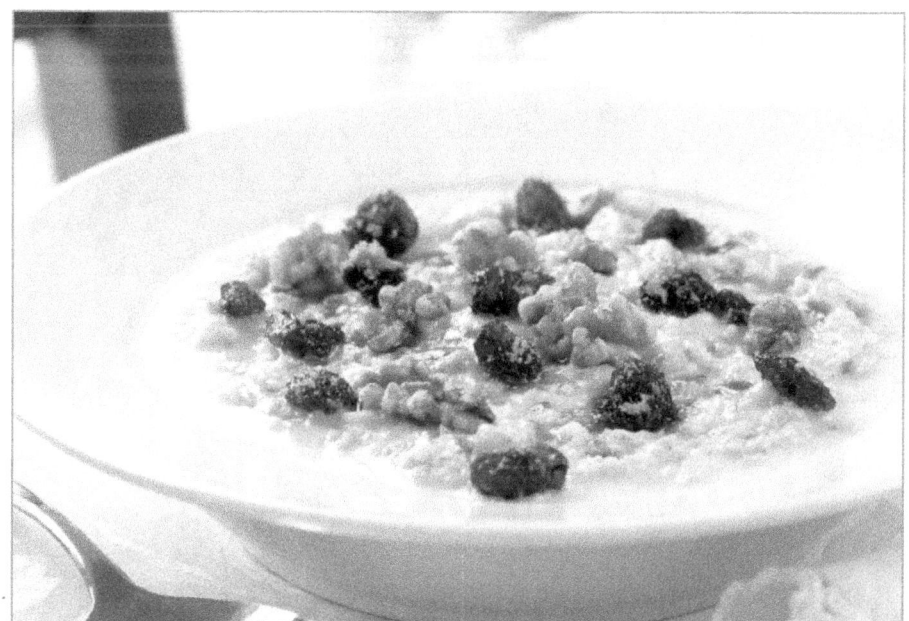

Ingredients:

- ½ cup of unsweetened coconut flakes
- ½ cup of chopped walnuts
- ¼ cup of slivered almonds
- 1 ½ tablespoons of hulled sunflower seeds
- 1 ½ tablespoons of hulled pumpkin seeds
- 4 cups of unsweetened coconut milk

Instructions:

1. Heat a dry skillet on the medium-low heat setting.
2. Add in the coconut, almonds, walnuts, pumpkin seeds and sunflower seeds.
3. Toast the ingredients for 2 to 3 minutes then transfer them to your food processor.

4. Add in your flaxseeds and blend the ingredients into a powder.
5. Transfer the powder to a large saucepan and stir in your coconut milk.
6. Heat the porridge on the medium heat setting until heated through. Serve warm.

Tomato Basil Omelet
Servings: 1

Ingredients:

- 1 medium vine-ripened tomato
- ¼ cup of chopped white onion
- 1 clove of garlic, minced
- 2 teaspoons of olive oil, divided
- 2 large eggs, whisked
- 1 scallion, sliced very thin
- Pepper and salt to taste
- 1 to 2 tablespoons of fresh basil, chopped

Instructions:

1. Heat up 1 teaspoon of your oil in a small skillet placed on the medium heat setting.
2. Add in the tomato, onion and garlic.
3. Cook the ingredients for 3 to 4 minutes until tender then spoon them off into a bowl.
4. Add in the rest of your oil to the skillet and heat it up to medium-high.
5. Stir together your eggs, scallion, pepper and salt.
6. Pour the eggs into your skillet and cook for about 2 minutes without stirring.
7. Lift the edges of the egg so the uncooked egg can spread.
8. When the egg is almost set, spoon your vegetables over half of the omelet.
9. Sprinkle on the basil then fold the omelet over your fillings.
10. Let the omelet cook for 30 seconds or so until it is completely set.

Maple Pecan Grain-Free Granola
Servings: 6 to 8

Ingredients:
- 1 cup of raw pecans
- ½ cup of slivered almonds
- ¼ cup of raw walnut halves
- ¼ cup of raw pumpkin seeds, hulled
- ¼ cup of chia seeds or flaxseeds
- ¼ cup of unsweetened coconut, shredded
- 1 ¼ teaspoon of ground cinnamon
- ½ teaspoon of salt
- 2 tablespoons of pure maple syrup
- 1 tablespoon of coconut oil, melted
- 1/3 cup of dried cranberries, chopped

Instructions:
1. Preheat the oven to a temperature of 300°F.
2. Combine all of the nuts and the seeds in a bowl.
3. Stir in your shredded coconut along with your cinnamon and salt.
4. Drizzle the ingredients with maple syrup and coconut oil.
5. Toss everything together until it is very well combined.
6. Line one of your baking sheets with a piece of parchment and spread out the granola out on it.
7. Bake for between 10 and 15 minutes until the granola is toasted – stir it halfway through.
8. Let the granola cool for a while then stir in the cranberries and serve.

Broccoli Onion Egg Muffins
Servings: 12

Ingredients:

- 1 teaspoon of coconut oil
- 1 small white onion, diced
- 1clove of garlic, minced
- 1 cup of frozen broccoli, thawed and chopped
- Pepper and salt to taste
- 12 large eggs, whisked well
- 2 tablespoons of chopped chives

Instructions:

1. Preheat your oven to a temperature of 350°F.
2. Spray the 12 cups in a regular muffin pan with cooking spray.
3. Melt the coconut oil in a skillet on the medium-high heat setting.
4. Add in the onions and garlic then season them with pepper and salt.
5. Cook the onions for 5 to 6 minutes until tender then take off the heat.
6. Stir the thawed broccoli into your onion mixture.
7. Spoon your vegetable mixture into your prepared muffin pan evenly.
8. In a bowl stir together your eggs and chives.
9. Pour the egg mixture into the muffin pan evenly then cook.
10. Cook for 20 to 25 minutes until the egg muffins are completely set.

Sweet Potato Cauliflower Hash
Servings: 4 o 6

Ingredients:

- 2 medium sweet potatoes, peeled and diced
- 1 head of cauliflower, cored and chopped up
- 1 medium yellow onion, diced
- ¼ cup of coconut oil, melted
- 1 tablespoon of paprika
- 1 teaspoon of dried oregano
- ½ teaspoon of cayenne
- Pepper and salt to taste

Instructions:

1. Preheat your oven to a temperature of 375°F.
2. Combine your sweet potatoes, cauliflower and onions in a bowl.
3. Drizzle in your coconut oil then toss with the paprika, oregano, and cayenne.
4. Season your mixture with some pepper and salt to taste.
5. Grease a rectangular glass baking dish with cooking spray.
6. Pour in your vegetable mixture and spread it out evenly.
7. Bake the hash for 30 to 35 minutes until your vegetables are tender.
8. Serve the hash warm with fried eggs, if desired.

Hormone Reset Soups and Salads

Warm Quinoa Veggie Salad
Servings: 6 to 8

Ingredients:

- 1 cup of uncooked quinoa, rinsed well
- 2 cups of chicken broth
- 1 tablespoon of coconut oil
- 1 small zucchini, peeled and diced
- 1 small red pepper, cored and diced
- 1 small yellow pepper, cored and diced
- 1 small yellow onion, diced
- ¼ cup fresh lemon juice
- 4 to 6 cups fresh chopped lettuce
- 1 cup cherry tomatoes, quartered
- Pepper and salt to taste

Instructions:

1. Stir together your quinoa and chicken broth in a large saucepan.
2. Bring your quinoa mixture to a boil over the high heat setting then cover it.
3. Lower the heat and simmer the quinoa for 15 to 20 minutes until it is tender.
4. Turn off the heat and fluff the quinoa with a fork – let it cool a little.
5. Heat your oil inside a large skillet set over the medium-high heat setting.

6. Stir in the zucchini, red pepper, yellow pepper and onion.
7. Cook for 6 to 8 minutes, stirring often, until the veggies are tender.
8. Stir the cooked quinoa and your lemon juice into the skillet and then transfer to a serving bowl.
9. Toss in the chopped lettuce and cherry tomatoes then season with pepper and salt to serve.

Dairy-Free Cream of Broccoli Soup
Servings: 6

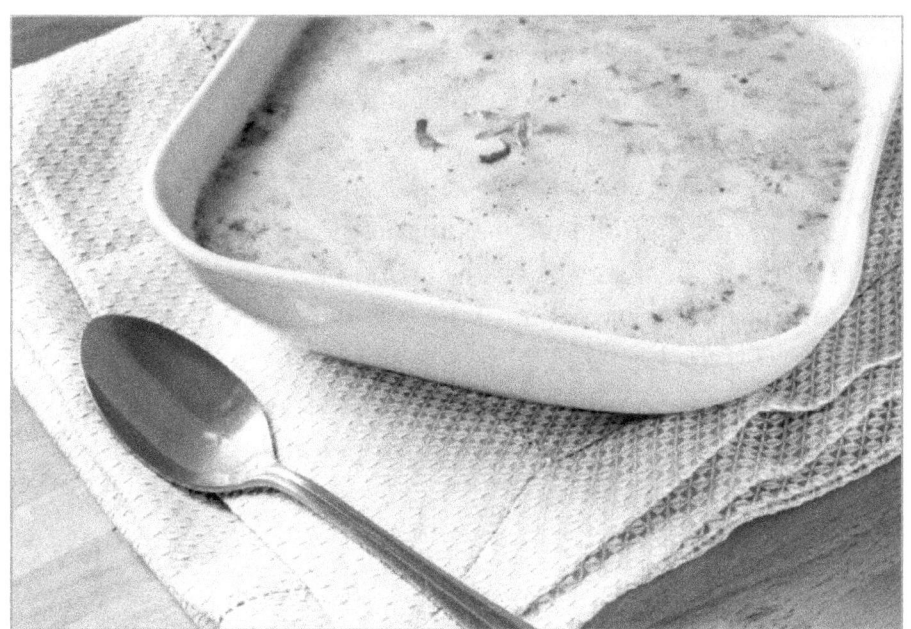

Ingredients:

- 2 large leeks, rinsed very well
- 4 cups of chopped up broccoli florets
- 1 medium white onion, chopped up
- 4 cups of low-sodium chicken broth
- 1 cup of canned coconut milk
- Pepper and salt to taste

Instructions:

1. Cut the roots and dark green parts off of the leeks and clean them well.
2. Slice the leeks lengthwise down the middle and then slice them up.
3. Place the leeks in a large-sized saucepan along with the broccoli and onion.
4. Add in your chicken broth and coconut milk.
5. Bring your ingredients to a boil on the high heat setting.
6. Lower the heat setting to low and simmer the ingredients for 20 minutes or just until the vegetables are nicely tender.
7. Turn off the heat and let your soup cool for a little while.
8. Puree the soup using an immersion blender until it is smooth.
9. Season your soup to taste with pepper and salt.

Cucumber, Red Onion, Dill Salad

Servings: 4 to 6

Ingredients:

- ½ medium red onion, sliced very thin
- Water, as needed
- 2 seedless cucumbers, halved lengthwise and sliced thin
- 2 to 3 tablespoons of fresh chopped dill
- ¼ cup of white wine vinegar
- 1 tablespoon of canned coconut milk
- Pepper and salt to taste

Instructions:

1. Place your red onions into a bowl and cover them with water – let them soak for around 10 minutes.
2. Drain your red onions and place them in a serving bowl with the cucumber and dill.
3. Whisk together the rest of your remaining ingredients into a dressing.
4. Pour the dressing over your prepared salad ingredients and toss them together well.
5. Chill your salad until you are ready to serve it.

Chilled Avocado Soup with Paprika

Servings: 6 to 8

Ingredients:

- 4 ripe avocadoes, pitted and chopped
- 3 medium shallots, chopped
- 3 ½ cups of chicken broth
- 1 cup of canned coconut milk
- Pepper and salt to taste
- Paprika, to serve

Instructions:

1. Combine your avocadoes and shallots into your food processor.
2. Add in your chicken broth and coconut milk.
3. Blend up the ingredients until the ingredients are smooth and very well blended.
4. Pour your blended up mixture into a bowl and season it with pepper and salt to taste.
5. Cover the bowl and chill it until the soup is cold.
6. Serve the soup cold sprinkled with paprika.

Dairy-Free Broccoli Salad

Servings: 4 to 6

Ingredients:

- ½ small red onion, sliced very thin
- Water, as needed
- 6 cups of fresh chopped broccoli florets
- ½ cup of sesame tahini
- ¼ cup of nutritional yeast
- 3 tablespoons of olive oil
- 2 ½ tablespoons of apple cider vinegar
- ½ teaspoon of dry mustard powder
- Pepper and salt to taste
- ¼ cups of thinly sliced almonds
- ¼ cup of toasted pumpkin seeds, hulled

Instructions:

6. Place your red onions in a bowl and cover with water – let them soak for about 10 minutes.
7. Put a metal steamer basket in a saucepan and add your broccoli.
8. Add an inch or so of water to the saucepan and then steam the broccoli for 4 to 5 minutes.
9. Drain your broccoli and then place it in an ice bath to chill.
10. Combine your tahini, nutritional yeast, olive oil, cider vinegar and mustard powder in a food processor.
11. Season with pepper and salt to taste then blend into a smooth dressing.

12. Drain your broccoli and your onions and place them in a serving bowl.
13. Add in your sliced almonds and pumpkin seeds then toss well with your dressing.
14. Chill the salad until you are ready to serve it.

Creamy Butternut Squash Soup
Servings: 4 to 6

Ingredients:

- 1 ½ tablespoons of coconut oil
- 1 large yellow onion, diced
- 2 small carrots, peeled and chopped
- 1 medium stalk celery, chopped
- 4 ½ cups of fresh chopped butternut squash
- 5 cups of chicken broth
- ½ teaspoon of fresh chopped thyme
- Pepper and salt to taste

Instructions:

1. Heat your oil inside a large pot on the medium-high heat setting.
2. Add in your onion, carrot and celery and then cook for about 4 to 5 minutes until the vegetables start to turn translucent.
3. Stir in your squash along with your chicken broth and thyme.
4. Season your soup with pepper and salt to taste then bring it to a boil.
5. Lower the temperature setting and simmer your soup for 30 minutes.
6. Turn off the heat and puree your soup using an immersion blender until it is very creamy.

Red Cabbage and Carrot Slaw
Servings: 6 to 8

Ingredients:

- 4 cups of thinly sliced red cabbage
- 2 cups of shredded carrots
- 4 green onions, sliced very thin
- 6 tablespoons of white wine vinegar
- 2 tablespoons of canned coconut milk
- 1 teaspoon of minced garlic
- ½ teaspoon of celery seed
- ¼ teaspoon of dry mustard powder

Instructions:

1. Combine your cabbage with the carrots and green onions in a large-sized bowl.
2. In a separate bowl, stir up together your remaining ingredients.
3. Drizzle the dressing over your salad ingredients and toss them well to combine them.
4. Chill the slaw until you are ready to serve it.

Hearty Curried Lentil Soup

Servings: 6 to 8

Ingredients:

- 2 tablespoons of olive oil
- 1 large yellow onion, chopped
- 2 small carrots, peeled and chopped
- 1 teaspoon of minced garlic
- 2 tablespoons of curry powder
- Pepper and salt to taste
- 1 cup of red lentils, rinsed well
- 4 cups of water

Instructions:

1. Heat your oil in a large saucepan on the medium-high heat setting.
2. Add in your onion and carrot and cook for 4 to 5 minutes until the vegetables start to turn translucent.
3. Stir in your garlic and curry powder then cook for another 2 minutes.
4. Season your soup with pepper and salt to taste then stir in your lentils and water.
5. Bring the soup to a boil on the medium-high heat setting.
6. Lower the temperature setting and simmer your soup for 30 minutes. Serve hot.

Spinach Salad with Avocado and Chickpeas

Servings: 4 to 6

Ingredients:

- 6 cups fresh chopped baby spinach
- 1 ½ cups of thinly sliced mushrooms
- ¼ cup of thinly sliced red onions
- 1 (15-ounce) can of chickpeas, rinsed and drained
- ½ teaspoon of turmeric
- ¼ teaspoon of garlic powder
- ½ cup of olive oil
- ¼ cup of red wine vinegar
- 1 tablespoon of Dijon mustard
- 1 clove of garlic, minced
- Pepper and salt to taste

Instructions:

1. Combine your spinach, mushrooms, and red onions in a salad bowl, tossing them together.
2. Drain the chickpeas well then add them to a dry skillet.
3. Heat the skillet on the medium-low heat setting and cook the chickpeas until they are toasted.
4. Toss the chickpeas with turmeric and garlic powder and set them aside.
5. Whisk up your remaining ingredients except for your avocado.
6. Toss your salad with your dressing and then garnish with sliced avocadoes and toasted chickpeas.

Southwestern Chicken Soup

Servings: 8 to 10

Ingredients:

- 1 tablespoon of olive oil
- ¾ lbs. of boneless skinless chicken, chopped
- 1 large yellow onion, chopped up
- 1 large red pepper, cored and chopped
- 1 tablespoon of minced garlic
- 1 tablespoon of chili powder
- 1 teaspoon of ground cumin
- 6 cups of chicken broth
- 1 (15-ounce) can of pinto beans, rinsed and drained
- 1 (14.5-ounce) can of diced tomatoes in juice
- 4 cups of fresh chopped kale
- 2 cups of frozen corn kernels

Instructions:

1. Heat your oil in a large saucepan on the medium-high heat setting.
2. Add in your chicken and cook for 4 to 5 minutes until it is lightly browned.
3. Transfer your chicken to a plate and reheat your saucepan.
4. Add in your onions, peppers, and garlic – cook them for 5 to 6 minutes until just they're tender.
5. Stir in your chili powder and cumin then cook it for about 30 seconds.
6. Add in your chicken broth, beans and tomatoes then bring your soup to a boil.

7. Lower the temperature and simmer the soup for 15 minutes.
8. Stir back into the soup the chicken along with the kale and corn.
9. Let the soup cook for 15 minutes then serve it hot.

Hormone Reset Snacks and Sides

Baked Zucchini Fritters
Servings: 12

Ingredients:

- 3 medium zucchini, shredded well
- 1 medium yellow onion, diced
- 2 to 3 tablespoons of chopped chives
- 1 teaspoon of minced garlic
- 1 cup of almond flour
- 2 large eggs, beaten well

Instructions:

1. Preheat your oven to a temperature of 400°F and grease up your muffin pan with cooking spray.
2. Spread your shredded zucchini on a clean towel then roll it up.
3. Wring out as much water from the zucchini as you can then put it in a bowl.
4. Stir in your onion, chives and garlic along with your almond flour and eggs.
5. When the mixture is thoroughly combined, press it into the muffin pan.
6. Fill the cups equally and bake the fritters for 25 minutes until the tops are browned.

Cocoa Cashew Butter Bars

Servings: 8 to 10

Ingredients:

- 12 ounces of 100% dark chocolate, chopped up
- 2 tablespoons of coconut oil
- 1 teaspoon of vanilla extract
- 1 ½ cups of xylitol, divided
- 1 ½ cups of natural cashew butter
- 1 cup of canned coconut milk

Instructions:

1. Melt the chocolate in a double boiler on the low heat setting.
2. When the chocolate is melted, stir in your oil, vanilla extract, and ½ cup of the xylitol.
3. Place a piece of parchment paper down in a baking dish.
4. Pour in the chocolate mixture and spread it evenly in the dish then freeze for 30 minutes.
5. Combine your cashew butter and coconut milk in a bowl with the rest of the xylitol.
6. Stir until well combined then spread it over the chocolate.
7. Cover the dish and freeze for 1 hour and then cut into squares to serve.

Lemon Garlic Hummus
Servings: 6 to 8

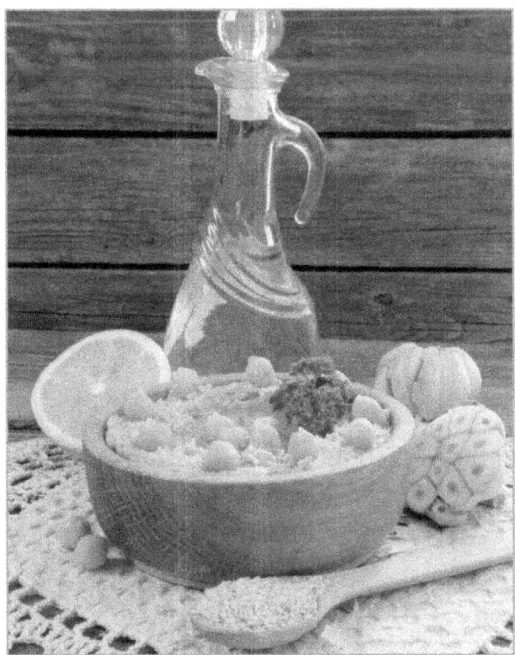

Ingredients:

- 2 cups of canned chickpeas, rinsed and drained
- ¾ cups of olive oil
- 2 to 3 tablespoons of lemon juice
- 1 teaspoon of fresh lemon zest
- 2 cloves of minced garlic
- Pepper and salt to taste

Instructions:

1. Drain your chickpeas well and place them in your food processor.
2. Add in your olive oil, lemon juice, lemon zest and garlic.
3. Blend the ingredients together until they are smooth.
4. Season your hummus with pepper and salt to taste.

Sesame Kale Chips

Servings: 4 to 6

Ingredients:

- 1 bunch of fresh kale
- 1 tablespoon of olive oil
- 1 teaspoon of sesame oil
- 1 tablespoon of sesame seeds

Instructions:

1. Preheat your oven to a temperature of 300°F and line your baking sheet with parchment.
2. Pat the kale dry with paper towels and trim away the thick stems.
3. Tear the kale into 3- or 4-inch pieces and place them in a bowl.
4. Toss the kale pieces with the olive oil and sesame oil.
5. Spread the kale leaves on the baking sheet and bake for 12 minutes.
6. Turn the baking sheet and bake for another 5 to 8 minutes until crisped.
7. Sprinkle the chips with sesame seeds and they are ready to serve.

Baked Sweet Potato Wedges

Servings: 6 to 8

Ingredients:

- 4 large sweet potatoes, peeled
- ½ cup of coconut oil
- 1 tablespoon of chili powder
- Pepper and salt to taste

Instructions:

1. Preheat your oven to a temperature of 400°F and line a baking sheet with parchment.
2. Cut the sweet potatoes into wedges then set them aside.
3. Melt your coconut oil inside a large skillet set over the medium-high heat setting.
4. Add in your sweet potatoes then toss in your chili powder and season with pepper and salt to taste.
5. Cook for 2 minutes then spread your sweet potato wedges on the baking sheet.
6. Bake the sweet potatoes for 20 to 30 minutes until they are browned and the edges are crisp.

Roasted Red Pepper Hummus

Servings: 6 to 8

Ingredients:

- 1 (15-ounce) can of canned chickpeas, rinsed and drained
- ½ cup of roasted red peppers, drained
- 6 tablespoons of tahini
- 4 to 5 tablespoons of fresh lemon juice
- 2 cloves of minced garlic

Instructions:

1. Drain your chickpeas well and place them in your food processor.
2. Add in your red peppers, tahini, lemon juice, and garlic.
3. Blend the ingredients together until they are smooth.
4. Season your hummus with pepper and salt to taste.

Dairy-Free Basil Pesto
Servings: 4

Ingredients:

- ½ cup of pine nuts, whole
- 2 cups of fresh basil leaves
- 1 tablespoon of minced garlic
- 1 to 2 tablespoons of olive oil, as need
- Pepper and salt to taste

Instructions:

1. Place your pine nuts into a dry skillet and heat them on medium-low.
2. Cook the pine nuts for a few minutes until they are toasted then remove from heat.
3. Place the pine nuts in your food processor along with the rest of your ingredients.
4. Blend up everything together until it is smooth and combined.
5. Season your pesto with some pepper and salt and serve immediately.

Baked Squash Fries
Servings: 4 to 6

Ingredients:

- 2 medium butternut squashes
- 1/3 cup of olive oil
- 1 teaspoon of paprika
- Pepper and salt to taste

Instructions:

1. Preheat your oven to a temperature of 425°F.
2. Line a baking sheet with parchment paper and set it off to the side.
3. Cut your butternut squash in half and scoop out all of the seeds.
4. Remove the peel from the squash and cut the flesh into sticks about ½-inch thick.
5. Toss your butternut squash fries with olive oil and spread them in the baking sheet.
6. Bake for 20 up to 25 minutes until the fries are nicely brown and crisp.
7. Season with paprika, pepper and salt to taste and serve warm.

Spicy White Bean Hummus

Servings: 6 to 8

Ingredients:

- 2 (15-ounce) cans white cannellini beans, rinsed and drained
- ¾ cups of sesame tahini
- 1 tablespoon of minced garlic
- ¼ cup of fresh lemon juice
- 1 teaspoon of ground cumin
- ½ cup of olive oil, more if needed
- Cayenne pepper, to taste

Instructions:

1. Drain your white beans then place them into a food processor.
2. Add in your tahini, garlic, lemon juice and cumin.
3. Blend up the ingredients until they are well combined.
4. Leave your food processor running and drizzle in your oil.
5. Once the hummus is smooth and blended, spoon it into a bowl.
6. Sprinkle with cayenne pepper to taste.

Easy Chia Seed Pudding
Servings: 4

Ingredients:

- 4 cups of canned coconut milk
- ¾ cups of chia seeds
- 1 teaspoon of vanilla extract
- Pinch of salt

Instructions:

1. Pour your coconut milk into a glass bowl.
2. Stir in your chia seeds along with your vanilla extract and salt.
3. Whisk the ingredients together very well then cover the bowl with plastic.
4. Chill the pudding for at least 2 hours and stir before serving.

Homemade Dairy-Free Cheese

Servings: 4 to 6

Ingredients:

- 2 cups of raw cashews
- ½ cup of nutritional yeast
- 1 tablespoon of minced garlic
- ½ cup of water, divided
- ¼ cup of lemon juice, divided
- 1 teaspoon of salt
- 2 to 3 teaspoons of fresh chopped parsley

Instructions:

1. Place your cashews in a bowl and cover them with water.
2. Let the cashews soak for at least 2 hours then drain them well.
3. Put your drained cashews into a food processor.
4. Add in your nutritional yeast, garlic and salt along with ¼ cup of water and 2 tablespoons of lemon juice.
5. Pulse these ingredients together until they are blended well.
6. Add in the rest of your lemon juice and some water, if needed, until it reaches the consistency that you like.
7. Spoon your cheese into a bowl and stir in your parsley to serve.

Almond Butter Fudge Cups

Servings: 18 to 24

Ingredients:

- 12 ounces of 100% dark chocolate, chopped up
- 2 tablespoons of coconut oil
- 1 teaspoon of vanilla extract
- 1 ½ cups of xylitol, divided
- 1 ½ cups of natural almond butter
- 1 cup of canned coconut milk

Instructions:

1. Melt the chocolate in a double boiler on the low heat setting.
2. When the chocolate is melted, stir in your oil, vanilla extract, and ½ cup of the xylitol.
3. Grease a 24-cup silicone mini muffin mold with cooking spray.
4. Pour in the chocolate mixture into the cups, filling them halfway, then freeze for 30 minutes.
5. Combine your almond butter and coconut milk in a bowl with the rest of the xylitol.
6. Stir until well combined then spread it over the chocolate mixture.
7. Freeze for 1 hour until firm then pop the fudge cups out of the mold to serve.

Hormone Reset Main Entrees

Coconut-Crusted Halibut Fillets
Servings: 4

Ingredients:

- 4 (6 to 8-ounce) boneless halibut fillets
- Pepper and salt to taste
- ½ cup of shredded coconut, unsweetened
- ¼ cup of almond flour
- ½ teaspoon of garlic powder
- 1 large egg, beaten
- Lemon wedges

Instructions:

1. Preheat your oven to a temperature of 350°F.
2. Season your halibut fillets with a little pepper and salt.
3. Combine your coconut and almond flour in a shallow dish with the garlic powder.
4. Beat the egg in another shallow dish.
5. Dip each fillet into the egg and then dredge it with the coconut mixture.
6. Place your fillets on a foil-lined baking sheet.
7. Bake the fillets for 12 to 15 minutes until the fish has just been cooked through.
8. Serve your fillets hot with wedges of lemon.

Sweet Potato Chickpea Curry

Servings: 4 to 6

Ingredients:

- 1 tablespoon of coconut oil
- 1 medium white onion, chopped
- 1 tablespoon of minced garlic
- 1 teaspoon of curry powder
- ½ teaspoon of ground turmeric
- ½ teaspoon of ground cumin
- ¼ teaspoon of dried coriander
- 1 (15-ounce) can of chickpeas, rinsed and drained
- 1 (14.5-ounce) can of diced tomatoes in juice
- 1 (14-ounce) can of light coconut milk
- 1 large sweet potato, peeled and chopped
- ½ cup of fresh chopped parsley

Instructions:

1. Heat your coconut oil in a large, deep skillet on the medium heat setting.
2. Ad your onion and garlic then cook for 4 to 5 minutes.
3. Stir in your spices and then cook them for 1 minute until very fragrant.
4. Add in your chickpeas, tomatoes, sweet potato and coconut milk.
5. Bring the mixture to a simmer and cook it for 30 to 45 minutes on the low heat setting until thick and hot.
6. Stir in your fresh chopped parsley and serve hot.

Cajun-Style Seared Scallops

Servings: 4

Ingredients:

- 2 tablespoons of coconut oil
- 1 large yellow onion, sliced thin
- 1 teaspoon of minced garlic
- 2 teaspoons of Cajun seasoning
- Pepper and salt to taste
- 1 ½ lbs. of fresh sea scallops, rinsed and patted dry

Instructions:

1. Melt the coconut oil in a cast-iron skillet on the high heat setting.
2. Add your onion and garlic then cook for 3 minutes.
3. Stir in your seasoning along with the pepper and salt.
4. Cook for 30 seconds then place your scallops in the skillet.
5. Cook for 2 to 3 minutes on each side until just cooked through.

Zucchini Pasta with Lemon Sauce

Servings: 4 to 6

Ingredients:

- 1 teaspoon of coconut oil
- 1 small yellow onion, chopped
- 1 teaspoon of minced garlic
- ¼ cups of canned coconut milk
- 2 to 3 tablespoons of fresh lemon juice
- 1 teaspoon of fresh lemon zest
- ½ cup of dairy-free cheese
- 2 medium zucchini, peeled

Instructions:

1. Heat your coconut oil in a deep skillet on the medium-high heat setting.
2. Add your onion and garlic then cook for 5 to 6 minutes until tender.
3. Whisk in your coconut milk and lemon juice along with the lemon zest.
4. Stir in your dairy-free cheese and cook the mixture until it starts to thicken.
5. Peel your zucchini into noodle-like threads using a vegetable peeler.
6. Toss the zucchini noodles into the lemon sauce and then cook for up to 2 minutes until just heated through.

Black Bean Mushroom Burgers

Servings: 6 to 8

Ingredients:

- 2 (15-ounce) cans of black beans, rinsed and drained well
- 1 cup of diced white mushrooms
- ½ cup of frozen spinach, thawed and squeezed to remove moisture
- 1 small yellow onion, diced
- 1 tablespoon minced garlic
- 1 ¼ cups of almond flour
- Pepper and salt to taste

Instructions:

1. Place your beans in a bowl and mash them a little bit with a fork.
2. Add in your mushrooms, spinach, onion, and garlic.
3. Stir in your almond flour then season the mixture with some pepper and salt to taste.
4. Shape the mixture into 8 even-sized patties using your hands.
5. Heat a large skillet on the medium heat setting and spray with cooking spray.
6. Add your patties and then cook them for 5 to 6 minutes on each side until they are browned.
7. Serve your burgers up on gluten-free buns with your favorite burger toppings.

Gluten-Free Crab Cakes

Servings: 6

Ingredients:

- 12 ounces fresh crabmeat
- 1 tablespoon of minced garlic
- 4 to 5 tablespoons of fresh chopped parsley
- ¾ cups of almond flour
- 1 ½ tablespoons of canned coconut milk
- 1 tablespoon of Dijon mustard
- 1 large egg, beaten well
- Pepper and salt to taste
- ¾ teaspoon of dried thyme

Instructions:

1. Flake your crabmeat into a bowl and add your garlic and parsley.
2. Stir in your almond flour, coconut milk, mustard and egg then season the mixture with pepper and salt to taste.
3. Add in your thyme and stir until well combined.
4. Shape your crab mixture into six even-sized patties about 3 ounces each.
5. Place the crab cakes on a parchment-lined baking sheet and chill for 1 hour, covered.
6. Heat a large skillet on the medium heat setting and spray with cooking spray.
7. Add your crab cakes and cook them for 4 to 5 minutes on each side until they are browned.

Seared Swordfish with Salsa

Servings: 4

Ingredients:

- 2 tablespoons of olive oil
- 4 (6 to 8-ounce) boneless swordfish steaks
- Pepper and salt to taste
- 2 small vine-ripened tomatoes, cored and diced
- ¼ cup of minced red onion
- ¼ cup of diced green pepper
- 2 tablespoons of fresh chopped cilantro
- 1 teaspoon of fresh lime juice
- Pinch of ground cumin

Instructions:

1. Heat your oil in a large skillet on the medium-high heat setting.
2. Season your swordfish steaks with pepper and salt to taste.
3. Place the swordfish in your skillet and cook for 2 to 3 minutes on each side until they are just seared.
4. Combine the rest of your ingredients inside a bowl, tossing them together.
5. Serve the swordfish steaks hot topped with the fresh salsa.

Cilantro Herbed Turkey Burgers
Servings: 6

Ingredients:

- 1 ½ lbs. of lean ground turkey
- ½ cup of almond flour
- ½ small red onion, diced fine
- ½ cup of fresh chopped cilantro
- 2 tablespoons of fresh chopped parsley
- Pepper and salt to taste

Instructions:

1. Combine your ground turkey with your almond flour and onions in a bowl.
2. Stir in your cilantro and parsley then season with pepper and salt.
3. Make sure the mixture is combined well then shape it into 6 patties.
4. Spray a large skillet with some cooking spray and heat it on medium-high.
5. Add your patties and cook them for 5 minutes on each side until they are cooked through.
6. Serve your turkey burgers on toasted gluten-free buns.
7. Add your favorite burger toppings like tomato, lettuce and onion.

Quick and Easy Ceviche

Servings: 4 to 6

Ingredients:

- 1 lbs. uncooked shrimp, peeled and deveined, chopped
- 1 small red onion, chopped fine
- 2 ½ cups of fresh lime juice
- 2 medium sized cucumbers, peeled
- 2 medium ripe avocadoes, pitted and diced
- 3 vine-ripened tomatoes, cored and diced
- Pepper and salt to taste

Instructions:

1. Combine your shrimp and onions in a bowl then add in the lime juice.
2. Toss them together then cover the bowl and chill it for 30 minutes.
3. Cut the cucumbers in half lengthwise and scoop out all of the seeds.
4. Chop the rest of the cucumber into small pieces.
5. Combine the cucumbers with the avocado and tomatoes in a bowl.
6. Stir in the shrimp and onion mixture then season with pepper and salt to taste.

Balsamic Portabella Burgers
Servings: 4

Ingredients:

- 4 large Portobello mushroom caps
- ¼ cup of olive oil
- ¼ cup of balsamic vinegar
- 2 tablespoons of lemon juice
- 2 teaspoons of Dijon mustard
- 1 teaspoon of minced garlic
- Pepper and salt to taste

Instructions:

1. Remove the stems from your mushroom caps and place them in a zippered freezer bag.
2. Whisk together your olive oil, balsamic vinegar, lemon juice, mustard and garlic.
3. Season the mixture with pepper and salt to taste.
4. Pour the marinade into the bag and seal it then shake to coat the mushrooms.
5. Let the mushrooms marinate for about 30 minutes at room temperature.
6. Preheat your grill and brush the grates using olive oil.
7. Place the marinated mushrooms on the hot grill and then cook them for 3 to 4 minutes per side.
8. Serve your mushroom burgers on toasted gluten-free buns with your preferred burger toppings.

Spaghetti Squash with Sautéed Veggies
Servings: 4 to 6

Ingredients:
- 1 large spaghetti squash
- Water, as needed
- 1 tablespoon of coconut oil
- 1 small yellow onion, chopped
- 1 teaspoon of minced garlic
- 1 small red pepper, cored and chopped
- 1 small zucchini, peeled and chopped
- Pepper and salt to taste

Instructions:
1. Preheat your oven to a temperature of 400°F.
2. Cut your spaghetti squash in half and scoop out all of the seeds.
3. Put the squash halves in a baking dish with the cut sides up.
4. Pour in about ½ inch of water into the dish then bake the squash for 30 to 45 minutes.
5. Let the squash cool a little bit until you can handle it.
6. Shred the squash with two forks into a bowl then set it aside.
7. Heat the oil in a large skillet on the medium-high heat setting.
8. Add your onions and garlic then cook them for 5 minutes.
9. Stir in your red pepper and zucchini then cook for 3 to 4 minutes until tender.
10. Add in your spaghetti squash and season with pepper and salt to taste.
11. Cook for 2 to 3 minutes they are until heated through then serve hot.

Conclusion

Please let me know your favorites- the review section of this book is an excellent place to share your experience with other readers.

I would love to hear from you!

To post an honest review, please visit:

http://amazon.com/author/kira-novac

DON'T FORGET YOUR FREE EBOOK

Irresistible Gluten Free Desserts, Snacks & Treats

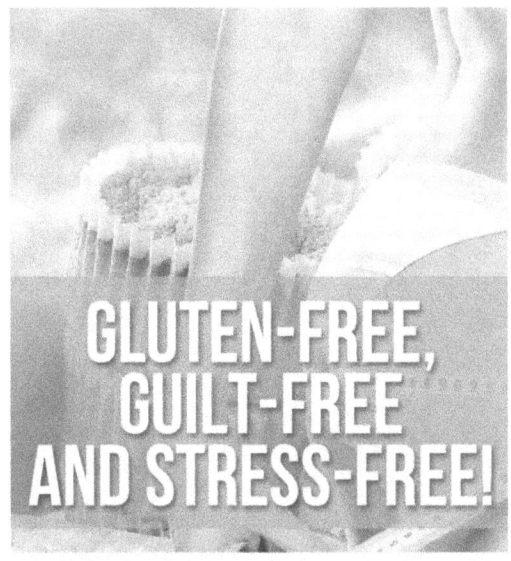

Download Link:

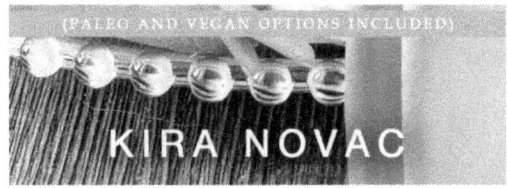

bit.ly/gluten-free-desserts-book

RECOMMENDED READING

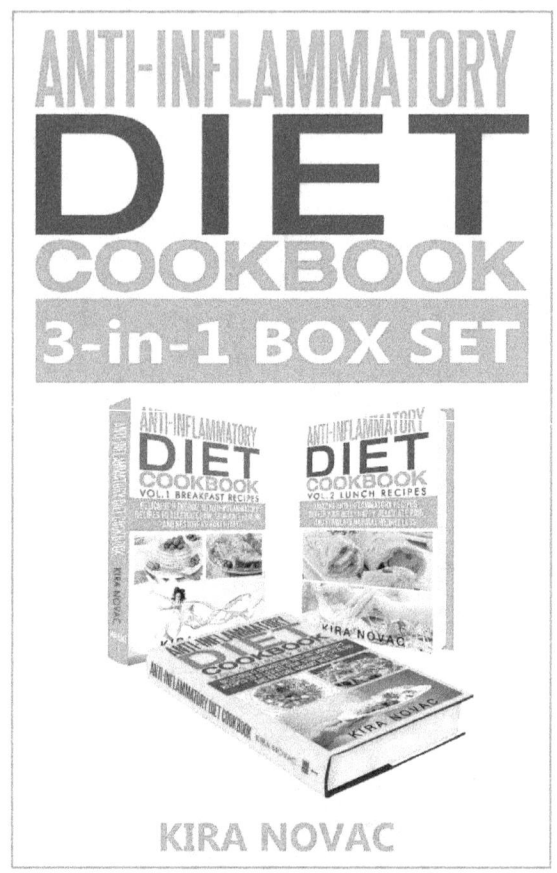

Amazon Book Page Link:

bit.ly/ai-box-set

RECOMMENDED READING

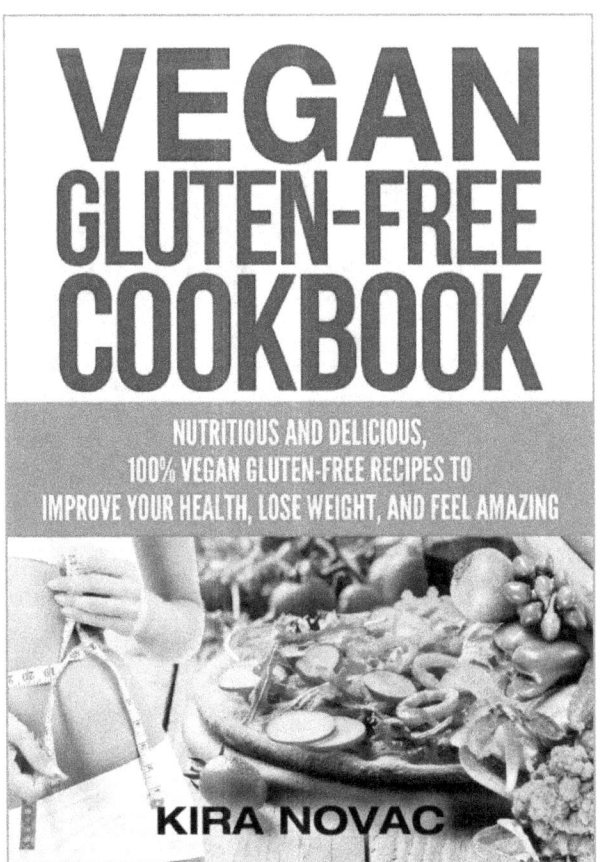

Amazon Book Page Link:

bit.ly/vegan-gluten-free

FOR MORE HEALTH BOOKS (KINDLE & PAPERBACK) BY KIRA NOVAC PLEASE VISIT:

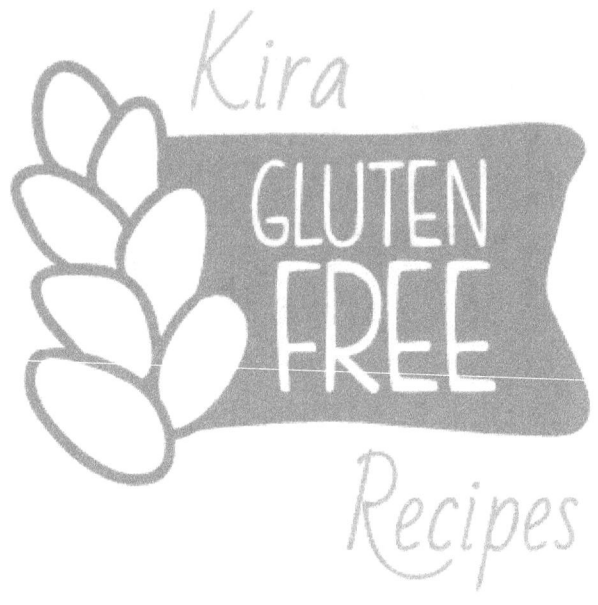

www.kiraglutenfreerecipes.com/books

Thank you for taking an interest in my work,

Kira and Holistic Wellness Books

HOLISTIC WELLNESS & HEALTH BOOKS

If you are interested in health, wellness, spirituality and personal development, visit our page and be the first one to know about free and 0.99 eBooks:

www.HolisticWellnessBooks.com

www.ingramcontent.com/pod-product-compliance
Lightning Source LLC
Chambersburg PA
CBHW072208100526
44589CB00015B/2430